Cram101 Textbook Outlines to accompany:

Foundations of Periodontics for the Dental Hygienist

Jill S Nield-Gehrig, 2nd Edition

A Content Technologies Inc. publication (c) 2012.

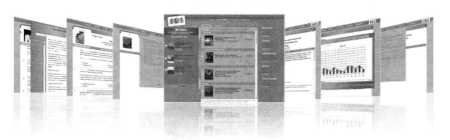

Learning System

Cram101 Textbook Outlines is a learning system. The notes in this book are the highlights of your textbook, you will never have to highlight a book again.

How to use this book. Take this book to class, it is your notebook for the lecture. The notes and highlights on the left hand side of the pages follow the outline and order of the textbook. All you have to do is follow along while your instructor presents the lecture. Circle the items emphasized in class and add other important information on the right side. With Cram101 Textbook Outlines you'll spend less time writing and more time listening. Learning becomes more efficient.

Cram101.com Online

Increase your studying efficiency by using Cram101.com's practice tests and online reference material. It is the perfect complement to Cram101 Textbook Outlines. Use self-teaching matching tests or simulate in-class testing with comprehensive multiple choice tests, or simply use Cram's true and false tests for quick review. Cram101.com even allows you to enter your in-class notes for an integrated studying format combining the textbook notes with your class notes.

Visit **www.Cram101.com**, click Sign Up at the top of the screen, and enter **DK73DW12578** in the promo code box on the registration screen. Your access to www.Cram101.com is discounted by 50% because you have purchased this book. Sign up and stop highlighting textbooks forever.

Foundations of Periodontics for the Dental Hygienist
Jill S Nield-Gehrig, 2nd

CONTENTS

Chapter 1. PART I: Chapter 1 - Chapter 10

Blood	Blood is a specialized bodily fluid that delivers necessary substances to the body's cells - such as nutrients and oxygen - and transports waste products away from those same cells.
	In vertebrates, it is composed of Blood cells suspended in a liquid called Blood plasma. Plasma, which constitutes 55% of Blood fluid, is mostly water (90% by volume), and contains dissolved proteins, glucose, mineral ions, hormones, carbon dioxide , platelets and Blood cells themselves.
Cementum	Cementum is a specialized calcified substance covering the root of a tooth. Cementum is excreted by cells called cementoblasts within the root of the tooth and is thickest at the root apex. Its coloration is yellowish and it is softer than enamel and dentin due to being less mineralized.
Gingiva	The Gingiva consists of the mucosal tissue that lies over the alveolar bone.
	Gingiva are part of the soft tissue lining of the mouth. They surround the teeth and provide a seal around them.
Periodontal ligament	The periodontal ligament, commonly abbreviated as the PDL is a group of specialized connective tissue fibers that essentially attach a tooth to the alveolar bone within which it sits. These fibers help the tooth withstand the naturally substantial compressive forces which occur during chewing and remain embedded in the bone.
	Another function of the PDL is to serve as a source of proprioception, or sensory innervation, so that the brain can detect the forces being placed on the teeth and react accordingly.
Periodontium	Periodontium refers to the specialized tissues that both surround and support the teeth, maintaining them in the maxillary and mandibular bones. The word comes from the Greek terms peri-, meaning 'around' and -odons, meaning 'tooth.' Literally taken, it means that which is 'around the tooth'. Periodontics is the dental specialty that relates specifically to the care and maintenance of these tissues.
	The following four tissues make up the Periodontium:
	· Alveolar bone

· Cementum

· Gingiva or gums

· Periodontal ligament

·

Ligament	In anatomy, the term Ligament is used to denote three different types of structures: · Fibrous tissue that connects bones to other bones. They are sometimes called 'articular larua', 'fibrous Ligaments', or 'true Ligaments'. · A fold of peritoneum or other membrane · The remnants of a tubular structure from the fetal period of life The study of Ligaments is known as desmology . Certain folds of peritoneum are referred to as Ligaments. Examples include: · The hepatoduodenal Ligament, that surrounds the hepatic portal vein and other vessels as they travel from the duodenum to the liver. · The broad Ligament of the uterus, also a fold of peritoneum. · The suspensory Ligament of the ovary

Chapter 1. PART I: Chapter 1 - Chapter 10

	Certain tubular structures from the fetal period are referred to as Ligaments after they close up and turn into cord-like structures:
	In its most common use, a Ligament is a band of tough, fibrous dense regular connective tissue comprising attenuated collagenous fibers.
Bone	Bones are rigid organs that form part of the endoskeleton of vertebrates. They function to move, support, and protect the various organs of the body, produce red and white blood cells and store minerals. bone tissue is a type of dense connective tissue.
Interdental	Interdental consonants are produced by placing the blade of the tongue (the top surface just behind the tip of the tongue) against the upper incisors. This differs from a dental consonant in that the tip of the tongue is placed between the upper and lower front teeth, and therefore may articulate with both the upper and lower incisors, while a dental consonant is articulated with the tongue against the back of the upper incisors.
	interdental consonants may be transcribed with both a subscript and a superscript bridge, as [nᵃíᵗ], if precision is required, but it is more common to transcribe them as advanced alveolars, for example [nÌŸ].
Mucogingival junction	A Mucogingival junction is an anatomical feature found on the intraoral mucosa. The mucosa of the cheeks and floor of the mouth are freely moveable and fragile, whereas the mucosa around the teeth and on the palate are firm and keratinized. Wherver the two tissue types meet is known as a Mucogingival junction.
Periosteum	Periosteum is a membrane that lines the outer surface of all bones, except at the joints of long bones. Endosteum lines the inner surface of all bones.
	Periosteum consists of dense irregular connective tissue.
Trigeminal nerve	The Trigeminal nerve is responsible for sensation in the face. Sensory information from the face and body is processed by parallel pathways in the central nervous system.
	The fifth nerve is primarily a sensory nerve, but it also has certain motor functions (biting, chewing, and swallowing).

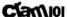

Chapter 1. PART I: Chapter 1 - Chapter 10

Dental implant	A dental implant is an artificial tooth root replacement and is used in prosthetic dentistry to support restorations that resemble a tooth or group of teeth. There are several types of dental implants. The major classifications are divided into osseointegrated implant and the fibrointegrated implant.
Gingival margin	The free Gingival margin is the interface between the sulcular epithelium and the epithelium of the oral cavity. This interface exists at the most coronal point of the gingiva, otherwise known as the crest of the marginal gingiva. Because the short part of gingiva existing above the height of the underlying Alveolar process of maxilla, known as the free gingiva, is not bound down to the periosteum that envelops the bone, it is moveable.
Mucosa	The mucous membranes (e; singular mucosa) are linings of mostly endodermal origin, covered in epithelium, which are involved in absorption and secretion. They line various body cavities that are exposed to the external environment and internal organs. It is at several places continuous with skin: at the nostrils, the lips, the ears, the genital area, and the anus.
Palate	The Palate is the roof of the mouth in humans and other mammals. It separates the oral cavity from the nasal cavity. A similar structure is found in crocodilians, but, in most other tetrapods, the oral and nasal cavities are not truly separate.
Junctional epithelium	The Junctional epithelium is that epithelium which lies at, and in health also defines, the base of the gingival sulcus. It attaches to the surface of the tooth with hemidesmosomes and is, on average, roughly 1 mm in width, constituting about one half of the biologic width. The Junctional epithelium lies immediately apical to the sulcular epithelium, which lines the gingival sulcus from the base to the free gingival margin, where it interfaces with the epithelium of the oral cavity.
Epithelium	Epithelium is a tissue composed of cells that line the cavities and surfaces of structures throughout the body. Many glands are also formed from epithelial tissue. It lies on top of connective tissue, and the two layers are separated by a basement membrane.

Chapter 1. PART I: Chapter 1 - Chapter 10

Alveolar process	The alveolar process is the thickened ridge of bone that contains the tooth sockets on bones that bear teeth. It is also referred to as the alveolar bone. In humans, the tooth-bearing bones are the maxilla and the mandible.
Mandible	The Mandible or inferior maxillary bone forms the lower jaw and holds the lower teeth in place. It also refers to both the upper and lower sections of the beaks of birds; in this case the 'lower Mandible' corresponds to the Mandible of humans while the 'upper Mandible' is functionally equivalent to the human maxilla but mainly consists of the premaxillary bones. Conversely, in bony fish for example, the Mandible may be termed 'lower maxilla'. The Mandible consists of: · a curved, horizontal portion, the body.
Teeth	Teeth are small, calcified, whitish structures found in the jaws (or mouths) of many vertebrates that are used to break down food. Some animals, particularly carnivores, also use Teeth for hunting or for defensive purposes. The roots of Teeth are covered by gums.
Cementoenamel junction	The Cementoenamel junction, frequently abbreviated as the CEJ, is an anatomical landmark identified on a tooth. It is the location where the enamel, which covers the crown of a tooth, and the cementum, which covers the root of a tooth, meet. The border created by these two dental tissues has much significance as it is usually the location where the gingiva attaches to a healthy tooth by fibers called the gingival fibers.
Dental pellicle	Dental pellicle is a protein film that forms on the surface enamel by selective binding of glycoproteins from saliva that prevents continuous deposition of salivary calcium phosphate. It forms in seconds after a tooth is cleaned. It is also protective to the tooth from the acids produced by oral microorganisms after consuming the available carbohydrates.
Osteoblast	Osteoblasts are mononucleate cells that are responsible for bone formation; in essence, Osteoblasts are sophisticated fibroblasts that express all genes that fibroblasts express, with the addition of the genes for bone sialoprotein and osteocalcin. Osteoblasts produce osteoid, which is composed mainly of Type I collagen. Osteoblasts are also responsible for mineralization of the osteoid matrix.

Chapter 1. PART I: Chapter 1 - Chapter 10

Osteoclast	An osteoclast is a type of bone cell that removes bone tissue by removing its mineralized matrix and breaking up the organic bone (organic dry weight is 90% collagen). This process is known as bone resorption. osteoclasts and osteoblasts are instrumental in controlling the amount of bone tissue: osteoblasts form bone, osteoclasts resorb bone.
Sulcular epithelium	The Sulcular epithelium is that epithelium which lines the gingival sulcus. It is apically bounded by the junctional epithelium and meets the epithelium of the oral cavity at the height of the free gingival margin. The Sulcular epithelium is nonkeratinized.
Gingivitis	Gingivitis around the teeth is a general term for gingival diseases affecting the gingiva (gums). As generally used, the term gingivitis refers to gingival inflammation induced by bacterial biofilms (also called plaque) adherent to tooth surfaces. gingivitis can be defined as inflammation of the gingival tissue without loss of tooth attachment (i.e.periodontal ligament).
Pathogenesis	The term Pathogenesis means step by step development of a disease and the chain of events leading to that disease due to a series of changes in the structure and /or function of a cell/tissue/organ being caused by a microbial, chemical or physical agent. The Pathogenesis of a disease is the mechanism by which a disease is caused. The term can also be used to describe the development of the disease, such as acute, chronic and recurrent.
Periodontitis	Periodontitis refers to a number of inflammatory diseases affecting the periodontium -- that is, the tissues that surround and support the teeth. periodontitis involves progressive loss of the alveolar bone around the teeth, and if left untreated, can lead to the loosening and subsequent loss of teeth. periodontitis is caused by microorganisms that adhere to and grow on the tooth's surfaces, along with an overly aggressive immune response against these microorganism.
Periodontal disease	Periodontal diseases are those diseases that affect one or more of the periodontal tissues: · alveolar bone · periodontal ligament · cementum · gingiva

While many different diseases affect the tooth-supporting structures, plaque-induced inflammatory lesions make up the vast majority of Periodontal diseases and have traditionally been divided into two categories:

· gingivitis or

· periodontitis.

While in some sites or individuals, gingivitis never progresses to periodontitis, data indicates that gingivitis always precedes periodontitis.

Investigation into the causes and characteristics of Periodontal diseases began in the 18th century with pure clinical observation, and this remained the primary form of investigation well into the 19th century. During this time, the signs and symptoms of Periodontal diseases were firmly established:

· Rather than a single disease entity, Periodontal disease is a combination of multiple disease processes that share a common clinical manifestation.

· The etiology (cause) includes both local and systemic factors.

· The disease consists of a chronic inflammation associated with loss of alveolar bone.

· Advanced disease features include pus and exudates.

· Essential aspects of successful treatment of Periodontal disease include initial debridement and maintenance of proper oral hygiene.

Periodontal pockets	Gingival and Periodontal pockets are dental terms indicating the presence of an abnormal gingival sulcus near the point at which the gums contact a tooth.

Chapter 1. PART I: Chapter 1 - Chapter 10

Contrary to what may be perceived by most people, the interface between a tooth and the surrounding gingival tissue is a dynamic place. The gingival tissue forms a crevice surrounding the tooth, similar to a miniature fluid-filled moat, within which food debris, both endogenous and exogenous cells, and chemicals float.

Periodontal pockets

Gingival and Periodontal pockets are dental terms indicating the presence of an abnormal gingival sulcus near the point at which the gums contact a tooth.

Contrary to what may be perceived by most people, the interface between a tooth and the surrounding gingival tissue is a dynamic place. The gingival tissue forms a crevice surrounding the tooth, similar to a miniature fluid-filled moat, within which food debris, both endogenous and exogenous cells, and chemicals float.

Gingival fibers

The Gingival fibers are the connective tissue fibers that inhabit the gingival tissue adjacent to the teeth and help hold the tissue firmly against the teeth. They are primarily composed to type I collagen, although type III fibers are also involved.

These fibers, unlike the fibers of the periodontal ligament, in general, attach the tooth to the gingival tissue, rather than the tooth to the alveolar bone.

The Gingival fibers accomplish the following tasks:

· They hold the marginal gingiva against the tooth

· They provide the marginal gingiva with enough rigidity to withstand the forces of mastication without distorting

· They serve to stabilize the marginal gingiva by uniting it with both the tissue of the more rigid attached gingiva as well as the cementum layer of the tooth.

Chapter 1. PART I: Chapter 1 - Chapter 10

Epidemiology	Epidemiology is the study of factors affecting the health and illness of populations, and serves as the foundation and logic of interventions made in the interest of public health and preventive medicine. It is considered a cornerstone methodology of public health research, and is highly regarded in evidence-based medicine for identifying risk factors for disease and determining optimal treatment approaches to clinical practice. In the study of communicable and non-communicable diseases, the work of epidemiologists ranges from outbreak investigation to study design, data collection and analysis including the development of statistical models to test hypotheses and the documentation of results for submission to peer-reviewed journals.
Pathogen	A Pathogen, 'I give birth to') an infectious agent, or more commonly germ, is a biological agent that causes disease to its host. There are several substrates and pathways whereby Pathogens can invade a host; the principal pathways have different episodic time frames, but soil contamination has the longest or most persistent potential for harboring a Pathogen. The body contains many natural orders of defense against some of the common Pathogens in the form of the human immune system and by some 'helpful' bacteria present in the human body's normal flora.
Prevalence	In epidemiology, the Prevalence of a disease in a statistical population is defined as the total number of cases of the disease in the population at a given time, or the total number of cases in the population, divided by the number of individuals in the population. It is used as an estimate of how common a condition is within a population over a certain period of time. It helps physicians or other health professionals understand the probability of certain diagnoses and is routinely used by epidemiologists, health care providers, government agencies and insurers.
Assessment	Educational Assessment is the process of documenting, usually in measurable terms, knowledge, skills, attitudes and beliefs. Assessment can focus on the individual learner, the learning community (class, workshop, or other organized group of learners), the institution, or the educational system as a whole. According to the Academic Exchange Quarterly: 'Studies of a theoretical or empirical nature addressing the Assessment of learner aptitude and preparation, motivation and learning styles, learning outcomes in achievement and satisfaction in different educational contexts are all welcome, as are studies addressing issues of measurable standards and benchmarks'.
Risk factor	In epidemiology, a Risk factor is a variable associated with an increased risk of disease or infection. Sometimes, determinant is also used, being a variable associated with either increased or decreased risk. Risk factors or determinants are correlational and not necessarily causal, because correlation does not imply causation.

Chapter 1. PART I: Chapter 1 - Chapter 10

Tooth loss	Tooth loss is when one or more teeth come loose and fall out. Tooth loss is normal for deciduous teeth (baby teeth), when they are replaced by a person's adult teeth. Otherwise, losing teeth is undesirable and is the result of injury or disease, such as mouth trauma, tooth injury, tooth decay, and gum disease.
Dental plaque	Dental plaque is biofilm (usually colorless) that builds up on the teeth. If not removed regularly by good oral hygiene measures, it can lead to dental cavities (caries) or periodontal problems . Plaque consists of microorganisms and extracellular matrix.
Biofilm	A biofilm is an aggregate of microorganisms in which cells are stuck to each other and/or to a surface. These adherent cells are frequently embedded within a self-produced matrix of extracellular polymeric substance (EPS). biofilm EPS, which is also referred to as 'slime,' is a polymeric jumble of DNA, proteins and polysaccharides.
Bacteroides forsythus	Bacteroides forsythus is a species of bacteria. It is sometimes equated with Tannerella forsythia. It is found in deep subgingival pockets and is associated with aggressive periodontitis.
Biofilm	A biofilm is an aggregate of microorganisms in which cells are stuck to each other and/or to a surface. These adherent cells are frequently embedded within a self-produced matrix of extracellular polymeric substance (EPS). biofilm EPS, which is also referred to as 'slime,' is a polymeric jumble of DNA, proteins and polysaccharides.
Facultative anaerobic bacteria	A facultative anaerobic organism is an organism, usually a bacterium, that makes ATP by aerobic respiration if oxygen is present but is also capable of switching to fermentation. In contrast, obligate anaerobes die in presence of oxygen. Some examples of Facultative anaerobic bacteria are Staphylococcus (Gram positive), Escherichia coli (Gram negative), Corynebacterium (Gram positive), and Listeria (Gram positive).

Chapter 1. PART I: Chapter 1 - Chapter 10

Fusobacterium nucleatum	Fusobacterium nucleatum is an oral bacterium, indigenous to the human oral cavity, that plays a role in periodontal disease. This organism is commonly recovered from different monomicrobial and mixed infections in humans and animals. It is a key component of periodontal plaque due to its abundance and its ability to coaggregate with other species in the oral cavity.
Periodontology	Periodontology is the branch of dentistry which studies supporting structures of teeth, and diseases and conditions that affect them.
	The supporting tissues are known as the periodontium, which includes the gingiva (gums), alveolar bone, cementum, and the periodontal ligament. The word comes from the Greek words peri meaning around and odons meaning tooth.
Immunodeficiency	Immunodeficiency is a state in which the immune system's ability to fight infectious disease is compromised or entirely absent. Most cases of Immunodeficiency are acquired ('secondary') but some people are born with defects in the immune system, or primary Immunodeficiency. Transplant patients take medications to suppress their immune system as an anti-rejection measure, as do some patients suffering from an over-active immune system.
Infection	An Infection is the detrimental colonization of a host organism by a foreign species. In an Infection, the infecting organism seeks to utilize the host's resources to multiply, usually at the expense of the host. The infecting organism, or pathogen, interferes with the normal functioning of the host and can lead to chronic wounds, gangrene, loss of an infected limb, and even death.
Tumor	A Tumor or tumour is the name for a neoplasm or a solid lesion formed by an abnormal growth of cells (termed neoplastic) which looks like a swelling. Tumor is not synonymous with cancer. A Tumor can be benign, pre-malignant or malignant, whereas cancer is by definition malignant.
Necrosis	Necrosis is the premature death of cells and living tissue. Necrosis is caused by factors external to the cell or tissue, such as infection, toxins, or trauma. This is in contrast to apoptosis, which is a naturally occurring cause of cellular death.
Bruxism	Bruxism is characterized by the grinding of the teeth and is typically accompanied by the clenching of the jaw. It is an oral parafunctional activity that occurs in most humans at some time in their lives. In most people, Bruxism is mild enough not to be a health problem.

Chapter 1. PART I: Chapter 1 - Chapter 10

Occlusal trauma	Occlusal trauma is a dental term that refers to the damage incurred when teeth are left in traumatic occlusion without proper treatment. When the maxillary and mandibular dental arches approach each together, as they do, for example, during chewing or at rest, the relationship between the opposing teeth is referred to as occlusion. If this occlusal relationship is not balanced properly it may result in pain, tenderness and even mobility of the affected teeth.
Tongue	The tongue is a muscle on the floor of the mouth that manipulates food for chewing and swallowing (deglutition). It is the primary organ of taste, as much of the upper surface of the tongue is covered in papillae and taste buds. A secondary function of the tongue is speech, in which the organ assists.
Retention	Retention can have the following meanings: · Retention basin, instance retaining (e.g. water in the ground) · In learning: it is the ability to retain facts and figures in memory (spaced repetition) · Grade Retention, in schools, keeping a student in the same grade for another year (that is, not promoting the student to the next higher grade with his/her classmates) · Retention period, in Usenet, the time a news server holds a newsgroup posting before deleting it as no longer relevant · Judicial Retention, in the United States court system, a process whereby a judge is periodically subject to a vote in order to remain in the position of judge · Urinary Retention, the lack or inability to urinate · Employee Retention, the ability to keep employees within an organization · Retention agent is a process chemical
Crown	

A Crown is a term (Crown) referring to a part of the head or of a hat, or to a head ornament or type of headgear for the highest rank in a socio-political hierarchy. It is etymologically related to the cognate currency units Krone and Krona.

· Crown ceremonial headgear

· Tiara, a type of Crown

· Ancient Egypt:

· Hedjet

· Deshret

· Pschent

· Ancient Rome:

· Civic Crown

· Grass Crown

· Naval Crown

· Mural Crown

· Consort Crown

· Coronation Crown

· Heraldic Crown

· Imperial Crown

· Royal Crown

· Commonwealth realms:

· The Crown, the legal embodiment of Executive Government in Commonwealth countries

· State Crown

· Crown of St. Stephen, Hungary's Holy Crown

· Papal Tiara or Triple Tiara, the papal Crown

· Triple Crown, a series of three major events that establishes dominance in a particular sport; see for list in various sports

· British Crown coin

· British half Crown coin

· Czechoslovak koruna, former Czechoslovakia

· Czech koruna, Czech Republic

· Danish krone, Denmark

· Estonian kroon, Estonia

· Faroese króna, Faroe Islands

· Hungarian korona, Hungary

· Icelandic króna, Iceland

· Slovak koruna, Slovakia

· Swedish krona, Sweden

· Crown, Inverness

· Crown Gardens, Gauteng, a suburb of Johannesburg, South Africa

· Crown Hill (various places)

· Crown North, Gauteng, a suburb of Johannesburg, South Africa

· Crown Point (various places)

· Crown College, University of California, Santa Cruz, a residential college

· Crown College (Minnesota), a small private college in St. Bonifacius, Minnesota

· Crown College , an unaccredited school with approximately 900 students

Chapter 1. PART I: Chapter 1 - Chapter 10

· Crown College (Washington), a small, for-profit, predominantly online college located in Tacoma, Washington.

· A Crown of sonnets is a group of related sonnets

· Crown an enemy of Spider-Man

· Diu Crône, an Arthurian romance

· The Crown a Swedish death/thrash band

· Crown the top of the head

· Crown the branching leaf-bearing portion of a tree

· Crown ether, a family of heterocyclic molecules

· Crown group, a group of living organisms

· Crown vetch, a plant

· Crown a dental treatment

· Crown a portion of a tooth

· Sahasrara, the Crown chakra in Hindu tradition

· Crown of Thorns, in Christianity, the headgear placed on Jesus before his execution

· Crown of Immortality, a literary and religious metaphor appearing in Baroque art.

Chapter 1. PART I: Chapter 1 - Chapter 10

· Tree of Life, The concept of a many-branched tree illustrating the idea that all life on earth is related.

· Keter, is the topmost of the Sephirot of the Tree of Life in Kabbalah

· Crown of the Andes, a religious Crown once used in Holy Week ceremonies in Popayan.

· Crown Castle, an American communications company

· Crown Equipment Corporation, a manufacturer of industrial lift trucks

· Crown Financial Ministries, a non-profit financial services entity

· Crown Holdings, a packaging products company

· Crown Hotel, Nantwich, a grade-I-listed 16th-century inn

· Crown International, amplifier and microphone manufacturer founded in 1947

· Crown International Pictures, a film production company

· Crown Limited, an Australian gaming and entertainment company established in 2007

· Crown Media, a media production company

· Crowne Plaza, a hotel chain

· Crown Paints, a British paint manufacturer

· Crown Publishing Group, a subsidiary of Random House

· Crown Records, a number of different record labels

· Crown Wallpaper, a British wallpaper manufacturer

· Crown Worldwide Group, a relocation company based in Hong Kong

· Crown an automobile built in Detroit, MI, in 1905

· Crown Coach Corporation, an American school bus manufacturer

· Toyota Crown, a model of Toyota car

· Crowned, as in the winner of a beauty pageant

· Crown glass, the name for high quality glasses used in optics or glazing

· Crown Lager, a beer brewed in Melbourne since 1919

· Lester Crown American businessman

· HMS Crown, the name of five ships of the Royal Navy and one planned one

· Norwegian Crown, a cruise ship

· Norwegian krone, a currency .

AIDS	Acquired immune deficiency syndrome or acquired immunodeficiency syndrome (AIDS) is a disease of the human immune system caused by the human immunodeficiency virus (HIV).
	This condition progressively reduces the effectiveness of the immune system and leaves individuals susceptible to opportunistic infections and tumors. HIV is transmitted through direct contact of a mucous membrane or the bloodstream with a bodily fluid containing HIV, such as blood, semen, vaginal fluid, preseminal fluid, and breast milk.
Assessment	Educational Assessment is the process of documenting, usually in measurable terms, knowledge, skills, attitudes and beliefs. Assessment can focus on the individual learner, the learning community (class, workshop, or other organized group of learners), the institution, or the educational system as a whole. According to the Academic Exchange Quarterly: 'Studies of a theoretical or empirical nature addressing the Assessment of learner aptitude and preparation, motivation and learning styles, learning outcomes in achievement and satisfaction in different educational contexts are all welcome, as are studies addressing issues of measurable standards and benchmarks'.

Chapter 1. PART I: Chapter 1 - Chapter 10

Osteoporosis	Osteoporosis is a disease of bone that leads to an increased risk of fracture. In osteoporosis the bone mineral density (BMD) is reduced, bone microarchitecture is disrupted, and the amount and variety of proteins in bone is altered. osteoporosis is defined by the World Health Organization (WHO) in women as a bone mineral density 2.5 standard deviations below peak bone mass (20-year-old healthy female average) as measured by DXA; the term 'established osteoporosis' includes the presence of a fragility fracture.
Aggressive periodontitis	Aggressive periodontitis describes a type of periodontal disease and includes two of the seven classifications of periodontitis:

· Localized Aggressive periodontitis

· Generalized Aggressive periodontitis
Aggressive periodontitis is much less common than chronic periodontitis and generally affects younger patients than does the chronic form.

The localized and generalized forms are not merely different in extent; they differ in etiology and pathogenesis.

In contrast to chronic periodontitis, primary features that are common to both LAP and GAP are as follows:

· except for the presence of periodontal disease, patients are otherwise healthy

· rapid loss of attachment and bone destruction

· familial aggregation

Moreover, Aggressive periodontitis often presents with the following secondary features:

· Amounts of microbial deposits are inconsistent with the severity of the periodontal tissue destruction |

· elevated proportions of Aggregatibacter actinomycetemcomitans, and in some cases, of Porphyromonas gingivalis as well

· phagocyte abnormalities

· hyperresponsive macrophage phenotype, including elevated levels of prostaglandin E_2 (PGE_2) and interleukin 1β

· progression of pathogenesis may be self limiting

The 1999 Consensus Report published by the American Academy of Periodontology permitted the subdivision of aggressive periodontal disease into localized and generalized forms based on enough individually specific features, as follows:

· Localized Aggressive periodontitis

· circumpubertal onset

· robust serum antibody response to infective agents: the dominant serotype antibody is IgG2

· localized first molar/incisor presentation

· Generalized Aggressive periodontitis

· usually affects patients under 30 years of age

· poor serum antibody response to infective agents

· pronounced episodic nature of periodontal destruction

· generalized presentation affecting at least 3 permanent teeth other than first molars and incisors

Severity of periodontal tissue destruction is subclassified in the same fashion as is chronic periodontitis.

Treatment generally involves mechanical therapy (non-surgical or surgical debridement) in conjunction with antibiotics.

Endodontic	Endodontics, from the Greek endo and odons (tooth), is one of the nine specialties of dentistry recognized by the American Dental Association, and deals with the tooth pulp and the tissues surrounding the root of a tooth. If the pulp (containing nerves, arterioles and venules as well as lymphatic tissue and fibrous tissue) has become diseased or injured, Endodontic treatment is required to save the tooth. .
Abscess	An abscess is a collection of pus (dead neutrophils) that has accumulated in a cavity formed by the tissue on the basis of an infectious process (usually caused by bacteria or parasites) or other foreign materials (e.g., splinters, bullet wounds, or injecting needles). It is a defensive reaction of the tissue to prevent the spread of infectious materials to other parts of the body. The organisms or foreign materials kill the local cells, resulting in the release of cytokines.
Malnutrition	Malnutrition is the insufficient, excessive or imbalanced consumption of nutrients. A number of different nutrition disorders may arise, depending on which nutrients are under or overabundant in the diet. The World Health Organization cites Malnutrition as the gravest single threat to the world's public health.

Chapter 1. PART I: Chapter 1 - Chapter 10

Gingival enlargement	Gingival enlargement, the currently accepted terminology for an increase in the size of the gingiva, is a common feature of gingival disease. This is strictly a clinical description of the condition and avoids the erroneous pathologic connotations of terms used in the past such as hypertrophic gingivitis or gingival hyperplasia. Gingival enlargement can be caused by a number of various stimuli, and 'treatment is based on an understanding of the cause and underlying pathologic changes.'
	The terms hyperplasia and hypertropy are not precise descriptions of Gingival enlargement because these terms are strictly histologic diagnoses, and such diagnoses require microscopic analysis of a tissue sample.
Toothpaste	Toothpaste is a paste or gel dentifrice used with a toothbrush to clean and maintain the aesthetics and health of teeth. Toothpaste is used to promote oral hygiene: it can aid in the removal of dental plaque and food from the teeth, aid in the elimination and/or masking of halitosis and deliver active ingredients such as fluoride or xylitol to prevent tooth and gum disease (gingivitis). Some dentist recommendations include brushing your teeth at least twice a day, if not more.

Periodontitis	Periodontitis refers to a number of inflammatory diseases affecting the periodontium -- that is, the tissues that surround and support the teeth. periodontitis involves progressive loss of the alveolar bone around the teeth, and if left untreated, can lead to the loosening and subsequent loss of teeth. periodontitis is caused by microorganisms that adhere to and grow on the tooth's surfaces, along with an overly aggressive immune response against these microorganism.
Aggressive periodontitis	Aggressive periodontitis describes a type of periodontal disease and includes two of the seven classifications of periodontitis:
	· Localized Aggressive periodontitis
	· Generalized Aggressive periodontitis Aggressive periodontitis is much less common than chronic periodontitis and generally affects younger patients than does the chronic form.
	The localized and generalized forms are not merely different in extent; they differ in etiology and pathogenesis.
	In contrast to chronic periodontitis, primary features that are common to both LAP and GAP are as follows:
	· except for the presence of periodontal disease, patients are otherwise healthy
	· rapid loss of attachment and bone destruction
	· familial aggregation
	Moreover, Aggressive periodontitis often presents with the following secondary features:
	· Amounts of microbial deposits are inconsistent with the severity of the periodontal tissue destruction
	· elevated proportions of Aggregatibacter actinomycetemcomitans, and in some cases, of Porphyromonas gingivalis as well

· phagocyte abnormalities

· hyperresponsive macrophage phenotype, including elevated levels of prostaglandin E_2 (PGE_2) and interleukin 1β

· progression of pathogenesis may be self limiting

The 1999 Consensus Report published by the American Academy of Periodontology permitted the subdivision of aggressive periodontal disease into localized and generalized forms based on enough individually specific features, as follows:

· Localized Aggressive periodontitis

· circumpubertal onset

· robust serum antibody response to infective agents: the dominant serotype antibody is IgG2

· localized first molar/incisor presentation

· Generalized Aggressive periodontitis

· usually affects patients under 30 years of age

· poor serum antibody response to infective agents

· pronounced episodic nature of periodontal destruction

· generalized presentation affecting at least 3 permanent teeth other than first molars and incisors

	Severity of periodontal tissue destruction is subclassified in the same fashion as is chronic periodontitis.
	Treatment generally involves mechanical therapy (non-surgical or surgical debridement) in conjunction with antibiotics.
Necrosis	Necrosis is the premature death of cells and living tissue. Necrosis is caused by factors external to the cell or tissue, such as infection, toxins, or trauma. This is in contrast to apoptosis, which is a naturally occurring cause of cellular death.
Occlusal trauma	Occlusal trauma is a dental term that refers to the damage incurred when teeth are left in traumatic occlusion without proper treatment.
	When the maxillary and mandibular dental arches approach each together, as they do, for example, during chewing or at rest, the relationship between the opposing teeth is referred to as occlusion. If this occlusal relationship is not balanced properly it may result in pain, tenderness and even mobility of the affected teeth.
Tumor	A Tumor or tumour is the name for a neoplasm or a solid lesion formed by an abnormal growth of cells (termed neoplastic) which looks like a swelling. Tumor is not synonymous with cancer. A Tumor can be benign, pre-malignant or malignant, whereas cancer is by definition malignant.
Chronic periodontitis	Chronic periodontitis is a common disease of the oral cavity consisting of chronic inflammation of the periodontal tissues that is caused by accumulation of profuse amounts of dental plaque.
	It is one of the seven destructive periodontal diseases as listed in the 1999 classification.
	In the early stages, Chronic periodontitis has few symptoms and in many individuals the disease has progressed significantly before they seek treatment. Symptoms may include the following:
	· Redness or bleeding of gums while brushing teeth, using dental floss or biting into hard food (e.g. apples) (though this may occur even in gingivitis, where there is no attachment loss)

· Gum swelling that recurs

· Halitosis, or bad breath, and a persistent metallic taste in the mouth

· Gingival recession, resulting in apparent lengthening of teeth.

| Periodontal disease | Periodontal diseases are those diseases that affect one or more of the periodontal tissues: |

· alveolar bone

· periodontal ligament

· cementum

· gingiva
While many different diseases affect the tooth-supporting structures, plaque-induced inflammatory lesions make up the vast majority of Periodontal diseases and have traditionally been divided into two categories:

· gingivitis or

· periodontitis.
While in some sites or individuals, gingivitis never progresses to periodontitis, data indicates that gingivitis always precedes periodontitis.

Investigation into the causes and characteristics of Periodontal diseases began in the 18th century with pure clinical observation, and this remained the primary form of investigation well into the 19th century. During this time, the signs and symptoms of Periodontal diseases were firmly established:

· Rather than a single disease entity, Periodontal disease is a combination of multiple disease processes that share a common clinical manifestation.

· The etiology (cause) includes both local and systemic factors.

· The disease consists of a chronic inflammation associated with loss of alveolar bone.

· Advanced disease features include pus and exudates.

· Essential aspects of successful treatment of Periodontal disease include initial debridement and maintenance of proper oral hygiene.

Periodontal disease	Periodontal diseases are those diseases that affect one or more of the periodontal tissues:

· alveolar bone

· periodontal ligament

· cementum

· gingiva

While many different diseases affect the tooth-supporting structures, plaque-induced inflammatory lesions make up the vast majority of Periodontal diseases and have traditionally been divided into two categories:

· gingivitis or

· periodontitis.

While in some sites or individuals, gingivitis never progresses to periodontitis, data indicates that gingivitis always precedes periodontitis.

Investigation into the causes and characteristics of Periodontal diseases began in the 18th century with pure clinical observation, and this remained the primary form of investigation well into the 19th century. During this time, the signs and symptoms of Periodontal diseases were firmly established:

· Rather than a single disease entity, Periodontal disease is a combination of multiple disease processes that share a common clinical manifestation.

· The etiology (cause) includes both local and systemic factors.

· The disease consists of a chronic inflammation associated with loss of alveolar bone.

· Advanced disease features include pus and exudates.

· Essential aspects of successful treatment of Periodontal disease include initial debridement and maintenance of proper oral hygiene.

Abscess

An abscess is a collection of pus (dead neutrophils) that has accumulated in a cavity formed by the tissue on the basis of an infectious process (usually caused by bacteria or parasites) or other foreign materials (e.g., splinters, bullet wounds, or injecting needles). It is a defensive reaction of the tissue to prevent the spread of infectious materials to other parts of the body.

The organisms or foreign materials kill the local cells, resulting in the release of cytokines.

Periodontium

Periodontium refers to the specialized tissues that both surround and support the teeth, maintaining them in the maxillary and mandibular bones. The word comes from the Greek terms peri-, meaning 'around' and -odons, meaning 'tooth.' Literally taken, it means that which is 'around the tooth'. Periodontics is the dental specialty that relates specifically to the care and maintenance of these tissues.

The following four tissues make up the Periodontium:

· Alveolar bone

· Cementum

· Gingiva or gums

· Periodontal ligament

·

Immunodeficiency	Immunodeficiency is a state in which the immune system's ability to fight infectious disease is compromised or entirely absent. Most cases of Immunodeficiency are acquired ('secondary') but some people are born with defects in the immune system, or primary Immunodeficiency. Transplant patients take medications to suppress their immune system as an anti-rejection measure, as do some patients suffering from an over-active immune system.
Assessment	Educational Assessment is the process of documenting, usually in measurable terms, knowledge, skills, attitudes and beliefs. Assessment can focus on the individual learner, the learning community (class, workshop, or other organized group of learners), the institution, or the educational system as a whole. According to the Academic Exchange Quarterly: 'Studies of a theoretical or empirical nature addressing the Assessment of learner aptitude and preparation, motivation and learning styles, learning outcomes in achievement and satisfaction in different educational contexts are all welcome, as are studies addressing issues of measurable standards and benchmarks'.
Exudate	An Exudate is any fluid that filters from the circulatory system into lesions or areas of inflammation. It can apply to plants as well as animals. Its composition varies but generally includes water and the dissolved solutes of the main circulatory fluid such as sap or blood.
Gingiva	The Gingiva consists of the mucosal tissue that lies over the alveolar bone. Gingiva are part of the soft tissue lining of the mouth. They surround the teeth and provide a seal around them.
Recording	Recording is a process of capturing data or translating information to a format stored on a storage medium often referred to as a record. Historical records of events have been made for thousands of years in one form or another. Amongst the earliest are cave painting, runic alphabets and ideograms.

Chapter 2. PART II: Chapter 11 - Chapter 20

- Periodontal screening examination - is a periodontal assessment used to
1) Determine the periodontal health status of the patient
2) Identify patients needing a more comprehensive periodontal assessment.
- PERIODONTAL SCREENING & RECORDING (PSR)

Chapter 2. PART II: Chapter 11 - Chapter 20

Tooth loss	Tooth loss is when one or more teeth come loose and fall out. Tooth loss is normal for deciduous teeth (baby teeth), when they are replaced by a person's adult teeth. Otherwise, losing teeth is undesirable and is the result of injury or disease, such as mouth trauma, tooth injury, tooth decay, and gum disease.
Outcome	In game theory, an outcome is a set of moves or strategies taken by the players, or their payoffs resulting from the actions or strategies taken by all players. The two are complementary in that, given knowledge of the set of strategies of all players, the final state of the game is known, as are any relevant payoffs. In a game where chance or a random event is involved, the outcome is not known from only the set of strategies, but is only realized when the random event(s) are realized.
Diagnostic test	A Diagnostic test is any kind of medical test performed to aid in the diagnosis or detection of disease. For example: · to diagnose diseases · to measure the progress or recovery from disease · to confirm that a person is free from disease A drug test can be a specific medical test to ascertain the presence of a certain drug in the body (for example, in drug addicts). Some medical tests are parts of a simple physical examination which require only simple tools in the hands of a skilled practitioner, and can be performed in an office environment. Some other tests require elaborate equipment used by medical technologists or the use of a sterile operating theatre environment.
Mucogingival junction	A Mucogingival junction is an anatomical feature found on the intraoral mucosa. The mucosa of the cheeks and floor of the mouth are freely moveable and fragile, whereas the mucosa around the teeth and on the palate are firm and keratinized. Wherver the two tissue types meet is known as a Mucogingival junction.

Chapter 2. PART II: Chapter 11 - Chapter 20

Bone	Bones are rigid organs that form part of the endoskeleton of vertebrates. They function to move, support, and protect the various organs of the body, produce red and white blood cells and store minerals. bone tissue is a type of dense connective tissue.
Cementoenamel junction	The Cementoenamel junction, frequently abbreviated as the CEJ, is an anatomical landmark identified on a tooth. It is the location where the enamel, which covers the crown of a tooth, and the cementum, which covers the root of a tooth, meet. The border created by these two dental tissues has much significance as it is usually the location where the gingiva attaches to a healthy tooth by fibers called the gingival fibers.
Lamina dura	Lamina dura is compact bone that lies adjacent to the periodontal ligament, in the tooth socket. The Lamina dura surrounds the tooth socket and provides the attachment surface with which the periodontal ligament joins to. An intact Lamina dura is seen as a sign of healthy periodontium.
Periodontal ligament	The periodontal ligament, commonly abbreviated as the PDL is a group of specialized connective tissue fibers that essentially attach a tooth to the alveolar bone within which it sits. These fibers help the tooth withstand the naturally substantial compressive forces which occur during chewing and remain embedded in the bone. Another function of the PDL is to serve as a source of proprioception, or sensory innervation, so that the brain can detect the forces being placed on the teeth and react accordingly.
Ligament	In anatomy, the term Ligament is used to denote three different types of structures: · Fibrous tissue that connects bones to other bones. They are sometimes called 'articular larua', 'fibrous Ligaments', or 'true Ligaments'. · A fold of peritoneum or other membrane · The remnants of a tubular structure from the fetal period of life The study of Ligaments is known as desmology . Certain folds of peritoneum are referred to as Ligaments.

Examples include:

· The hepatoduodenal Ligament, that surrounds the hepatic portal vein and other vessels as they travel from the duodenum to the liver.

· The broad Ligament of the uterus, also a fold of peritoneum.

· The suspensory Ligament of the ovary
Certain tubular structures from the fetal period are referred to as Ligaments after they close up and turn into cord-like structures:

In its most common use, a Ligament is a band of tough, fibrous dense regular connective tissue comprising attenuated collagenous fibers.

Periodontal pockets	Gingival and Periodontal pockets are dental terms indicating the presence of an abnormal gingival sulcus near the point at which the gums contact a tooth.
	Contrary to what may be perceived by most people, the interface between a tooth and the surrounding gingival tissue is a dynamic place. The gingival tissue forms a crevice surrounding the tooth, similar to a miniature fluid-filled moat, within which food debris, both endogenous and exogenous cells, and chemicals float.
Periodontal pockets	Gingival and Periodontal pockets are dental terms indicating the presence of an abnormal gingival sulcus near the point at which the gums contact a tooth.
	Contrary to what may be perceived by most people, the interface between a tooth and the surrounding gingival tissue is a dynamic place. The gingival tissue forms a crevice surrounding the tooth, similar to a miniature fluid-filled moat, within which food debris, both endogenous and exogenous cells, and chemicals float.

Chapter 2. PART II: Chapter 11 - Chapter 20

Assessment	Educational Assessment is the process of documenting, usually in measurable terms, knowledge, skills, attitudes and beliefs. Assessment can focus on the individual learner, the learning community (class, workshop, or other organized group of learners), the institution, or the educational system as a whole. According to the Academic Exchange Quarterly: 'Studies of a theoretical or empirical nature addressing the Assessment of learner aptitude and preparation, motivation and learning styles, learning outcomes in achievement and satisfaction in different educational contexts are all welcome, as are studies addressing issues of measurable standards and benchmarks'.
Linear gingival erythema	Linear gingival erythema is a periodontal disorder diagnosed based on distinct clinical characteristics. It was originally thought that Linear gingival erythema was directly associated with HIV, and it was thus called HIV-associated gingivitis (HIV-G). Later research confirmed that Linear gingival erythema occurs in HIV negative immunocompromised patients, and it was thus renamed.
Erythema	Erythema is redness of the skin, caused by congestion of the capillaries in the lower layers of the skin. It occurs with any skin injury, infection, or inflammation. Erythema disappears on finger pressure (blanching), while purpura or bleeding in the skin and pigmentation do not.
Blood	Blood is a specialized bodily fluid that delivers necessary substances to the body's cells - such as nutrients and oxygen - and transports waste products away from those same cells. In vertebrates, it is composed of Blood cells suspended in a liquid called Blood plasma. Plasma, which constitutes 55% of Blood fluid, is mostly water (90% by volume), and contains dissolved proteins, glucose, mineral ions, hormones, carbon dioxide , platelets and Blood cells themselves.
Contraindication	A Contraindication is a condition or factor that speaks against a certain measure. It is mostly used in medicine, with regard to factors that increase the risks involved in using a particular drug, carrying out a medical procedure, or engaging in a particular activity. Some Contraindications are absolute, meaning that there are no reasonable circumstances for undertaking a course of action.

Chapter 2. PART II: Chapter 11 - Chapter 20

Case series	A Case series is a medical research study that tracks patients with a known exposure given similar treatment or examines their medical records for exposure and outcome.
	A Case series can be retrospective or prospective and usually involves a smaller number of patients than more powerful case-control studies or randomized controlled trials.
	A Case series is a type of observational study.
Cohort study	A Cohort study or panel study is a form of longitudinal study (a type of observational study) used in medicine, actuarial science and ecology. It is one type of study design and should be compared with a cross-sectional study.
	A cohort is a group of people who share a common characteristic or experience within a defined period (e.g.
Collaboration	Collaboration is a recursive process where two or more people or organizations work together in an intersection of common goals -- for example, an intellectual endeavor that is creative in nature--by sharing knowledge, learning and building consensus. Most Collaboration requires leadership, although the form of leadership can be social within a decentralized and egalitarian group. In particular, teams that work collaboratively can obtain greater resources, recognition and reward when facing competition for finite resources.
Symptom	A Symptom is a departure from normal function or feeling which is noticed by a patient, indicating the presence of disease or abnormality. A Symptom is subjective, observed by the patient, and not measured.
	A Symptom may not be a malady, for example Symptoms of pregnancy.
Dental implant	A dental implant is an artificial tooth root replacement and is used in prosthetic dentistry to support restorations that resemble a tooth or group of teeth.
	There are several types of dental implants. The major classifications are divided into osseointegrated implant and the fibrointegrated implant.

Chapter 2. PART II: Chapter 11 - Chapter 20

Debridement	In oral hygiene and dentistry, Debridement refers to the removal of plaque and calculus that have accumulated on the teeth. Debridement in this case may be performed using ultrasonic instruments, which fracture the calculus, thereby facilitating its removal, as well as hand tools, including periodontal scaler and curettes, or through the use of chemicals such as hydrogen peroxide.
Epithelium	Epithelium is a tissue composed of cells that line the cavities and surfaces of structures throughout the body. Many glands are also formed from epithelial tissue. It lies on top of connective tissue, and the two layers are separated by a basement membrane.
Junctional epithelium	The Junctional epithelium is that epithelium which lies at, and in health also defines, the base of the gingival sulcus. It attaches to the surface of the tooth with hemidesmosomes and is, on average, roughly 1 mm in width, constituting about one half of the biologic width.
	The Junctional epithelium lies immediately apical to the sulcular epithelium, which lines the gingival sulcus from the base to the free gingival margin, where it interfaces with the epithelium of the oral cavity.
Smear layer	The Smear layer is a layer of microcrystalline and organic particle debris spread on root canal walls after root canal instrumentation.
	Early studies of dentinal walls after cavity preparation performed by Brännström and Johnson (1974) showed a thin layer of debris that was 2 to 5 microns thick.
	In 1975 McComb and Smith first described the Smear layer after observing an amorphous layer of debris with an irregular and granular surface on instrumented dentinal walls using SEM.
Dental implant	A dental implant is an artificial tooth root replacement and is used in prosthetic dentistry to support restorations that resemble a tooth or group of teeth.
	There are several types of dental implants. The major classifications are divided into osseointegrated implant and the fibrointegrated implant.

Chapter 2. PART II: Chapter 11 - Chapter 20

Root planing	The objective of scaling and root planing, otherwise known as conventional periodontal therapy or non-surgical periodontal therapy, is to remove or eliminate the etiologic agents which cause inflammation: dental plaque, its products and calculus, thus helping to establish a periodontium that is free of disease.
	Periodontal scaling procedures 'include the removal of plaque, calculus and stain from the crown and root surfaces of teeth, whereas root planing is a specific treatment that removes the roughened cementum and surface dentin that is impregnated with calculus, microorganisms and their toxins.'
	Scaling and root planing are often referred to as deep cleaning, and may be performed using a number of dental tools, including ultrasonic instruments and hand instruments, such as periodontal scalers and curettes.
	Removal of adherent plaque and calculus with hand instruments can also be performed on patients without periodontal disease.
Tongue	The tongue is a muscle on the floor of the mouth that manipulates food for chewing and swallowing (deglutition). It is the primary organ of taste, as much of the upper surface of the tongue is covered in papillae and taste buds. A secondary function of the tongue is speech, in which the organ assists.
Interdental	Interdental consonants are produced by placing the blade of the tongue (the top surface just behind the tip of the tongue) against the upper incisors. This differs from a dental consonant in that the tip of the tongue is placed between the upper and lower front teeth, and therefore may articulate with both the upper and lower incisors, while a dental consonant is articulated with the tongue against the back of the upper incisors.
	interdental consonants may be transcribed with both a subscript and a superscript bridge, as [n̪ᵃ‡], if precision is required, but it is more common to transcribe them as advanced alveolars, for example [n̠Ÿ].

Health promotion	Health promotion has been defined by the World Health Organization's 2005 Bangkok Charter for Health promotion in a Globalized World as 'the process of enabling people to increase control over their health and its determinants, and thereby improve their health'. The primary means of Health promotion occur through developing healthy public policy that addresses the prerequisities of health such as income, housing, food security, employment, and quality working conditions. There is a tendency among public health officials and governments--and this is especially the case in liberal nations such as Canada and the USA--to reduce Health promotion to health education and social marketing focused on changing behavioral risk factors.
Preparation	Preparations is the fourth full-length album by Prefuse 73, released on October 23, 2007 on Warp Records . Unlike the 2006 EP Security Screenings, Preparations is considered the proper follow-up to 2005's collaboration-heavy Surrounded by Silence. In contrast to that album, Preparations features only one guest vocalist.
Osteoporosis	Osteoporosis is a disease of bone that leads to an increased risk of fracture. In osteoporosis the bone mineral density (BMD) is reduced, bone microarchitecture is disrupted, and the amount and variety of proteins in bone is altered. osteoporosis is defined by the World Health Organization (WHO) in women as a bone mineral density 2.5 standard deviations below peak bone mass (20-year-old healthy female average) as measured by DXA; the term 'established osteoporosis' includes the presence of a fragility fracture.
Gingivitis	Gingivitis around the teeth is a general term for gingival diseases affecting the gingiva (gums). As generally used, the term gingivitis refers to gingival inflammation induced by bacterial biofilms (also called plaque) adherent to tooth surfaces.

gingivitis can be defined as inflammation of the gingival tissue without loss of tooth attachment (i.e.periodontal ligament). |

Crown

A Crown is a term (Crown) referring to a part of the head or of a hat, or to a head ornament or type of headgear for the highest rank in a socio-political hierarchy. It is etymologically related to the cognate currency units Krone and Krona.

· Crown ceremonial headgear

· Tiara, a type of Crown

· Ancient Egypt:

· Hedjet

· Deshret

· Pschent

· Ancient Rome:

· Civic Crown

· Grass Crown

· Naval Crown

· Mural Crown

· Consort Crown

· Coronation Crown

· Heraldic Crown

· Imperial Crown

· Royal Crown

· Commonwealth realms:

· The Crown, the legal embodiment of Executive Government in Commonwealth countries

· State Crown

· Crown of St. Stephen, Hungary's Holy Crown

· Papal Tiara or Triple Tiara, the papal Crown

· Triple Crown, a series of three major events that establishes dominance in a particular sport; see for list in various sports

· Crown College (Washington), a small, for-profit, predominantly online college located in Tacoma, Washington.

· A Crown of sonnets is a group of related sonnets

· Crown an enemy of Spider-Man

· Diu Crône, an Arthurian romance

· The Crown a Swedish death/thrash band

· Crown the top of the head

· Crown the branching leaf-bearing portion of a tree

· Crown ether, a family of heterocyclic molecules

· Crown group, a group of living organisms

· Crown vetch, a plant

· Crown a dental treatment

· Crown a portion of a tooth

· Sahasrara, the Crown chakra in Hindu tradition

· Crown of Thorns, in Christianity, the headgear placed on Jesus before his execution

· Crown of Immortality, a literary and religious metaphor appearing in Baroque art.

· Tree of Life, The concept of a many-branched tree illustrating the idea that all life on earth is related.

· Keter, is the topmost of the Sephirot of the Tree of Life in Kabbalah

· Crown of the Andes, a religious Crown once used in Holy Week ceremonies in Popayan.

· Crown Castle, an American communications company

· Crown Equipment Corporation, a manufacturer of industrial lift trucks

· Crown Financial Ministries, a non-profit financial services entity

· Crown Holdings, a packaging products company

· Crown Hotel, Nantwich, a grade-I-listed 16th-century inn

· Crown International, amplifier and microphone manufacturer founded in 1947

· Crown International Pictures, a film production company

· Crown Limited, an Australian gaming and entertainment company established in 2007

· Crown Media, a media production company

· Crowne Plaza, a hotel chain

· Crown Paints, a British paint manufacturer

· Crown Publishing Group, a subsidiary of Random House

· Crown Records, a number of different record labels

· Crown Wallpaper, a British wallpaper manufacturer

· Crown Worldwide Group, a relocation company based in Hong Kong

· Crown an automobile built in Detroit, MI, in 1905

· Crown Coach Corporation, an American school bus manufacturer

· Toyota Crown, a model of Toyota car

· Crowned, as in the winner of a beauty pageant

· Crown glass, the name for high quality glasses used in optics or glazing

· Crown Lager, a beer brewed in Melbourne since 1919

· Lester Crown American businessman

· HMS Crown, the name of five ships of the Royal Navy and one planned one

· Norwegian Crown, a cruise ship

· Norwegian krone, a currency .

Crown lengthening	Crown lengthening is a surgical procedure performed by a dentist to expose a greater amount of tooth structure for the purpose of subsequently restoring the tooth prosthetically. This is done by incising the gingival tissue around a tooth and, after temporarily displacing the soft tissue, predictably removing a given height of alveolar bone from the circumference of the tooth or teeth being operated on. While many general dentists perform this procedure, they frequently refer such cases to periodontists.
Dental implant	A dental implant is an artificial tooth root replacement and is used in prosthetic dentistry to support restorations that resemble a tooth or group of teeth. There are several types of dental implants. The major classifications are divided into osseointegrated implant and the fibrointegrated implant.
Epithelium	Epithelium is a tissue composed of cells that line the cavities and surfaces of structures throughout the body. Many glands are also formed from epithelial tissue. It lies on top of connective tissue, and the two layers are separated by a basement membrane.

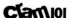

Chapter 3. PART III: Chapter 21 - Chapter 30

Gingival graft	A Gingival graft is a generic name for any of a number of surgical periodontal procedures whose combined aim is to cover an area of exposed tooth root surface with grafted oral tissue. The covering of exposed root surfaces accomplishes a number of objectives: the prevention of further root exposure, decreased or eliminated sensitivity, decreased susceptibility to root caries and improved cosmetic. These procedures are usually performed by a dental specialist in the field of gingival tissue, known as a periodontist, but may be performed by a general dentist having training in these procedures.
Gingivectomy	A gingivectomy is a periodontal surgical procedure which includes the removal of gingival tissue in order to achieve a more aesthetic appearance and/or functional contour. Gingivectomies are frequently performed using electrosurgery to cauterize away the undesired gum tissue.
Guided tissue regeneration	Guided bone regeneration or GBR, and guided tissue regeneration are surgical procedures that utilize barrier membranes to direct the growth of new bone and soft tissue at sites having insufficient volumes or dimensions for proper function, esthetics or prosthetic restoration. GBR is similar to guided tissue regeneration but is focused on development of hard tissues instead of soft tissues of periodontal attachment. At present, guided bone regeneration is predominantly applied in the oral cavity to support new hard tissue growth on an alveolar ridge to allow stable placement of dental implants.
Junctional epithelium	The Junctional epithelium is that epithelium which lies at, and in health also defines, the base of the gingival sulcus. It attaches to the surface of the tooth with hemidesmosomes and is, on average, roughly 1 mm in width, constituting about one half of the biologic width. The Junctional epithelium lies immediately apical to the sulcular epithelium, which lines the gingival sulcus from the base to the free gingival margin, where it interfaces with the epithelium of the oral cavity.
Plastic	Plastic is the general term for a wide range of synthetic or semi-synthetic organic amorphous solid materials used in the manufacture of industrial products. Plastics are typically polymers of high molecular mass, and may contain other substances to improve performance and/or reduce costs. Monomers of Plastic are either natural or synthetic organic compounds.

Repair	Maintenance, repair, and operations (MRO) involves fixing any sort of mechanical or electrical device should it become out of order or broken (known as repair, unscheduled or casualty maintenance). It also includes performing routine actions which keep the device in working order (known as scheduled maintenance) or prevent trouble from arising (preventive maintenance). MRO may be defined as, 'All actions which have the objective of retaining or restoring an item in or to a state in which it can perform its required function.
Bone	Bones are rigid organs that form part of the endoskeleton of vertebrates. They function to move, support, and protect the various organs of the body, produce red and white blood cells and store minerals. bone tissue is a type of dense connective tissue.
Contraindication	A Contraindication is a condition or factor that speaks against a certain measure. It is mostly used in medicine, with regard to factors that increase the risks involved in using a particular drug, carrying out a medical procedure, or engaging in a particular activity. Some Contraindications are absolute, meaning that there are no reasonable circumstances for undertaking a course of action.
Gingivitis	Gingivitis around the teeth is a general term for gingival diseases affecting the gingiva (gums). As generally used, the term gingivitis refers to gingival inflammation induced by bacterial biofilms (also called plaque) adherent to tooth surfaces. gingivitis can be defined as inflammation of the gingival tissue without loss of tooth attachment (i.e.periodontal ligament).
Periodontium	Periodontium refers to the specialized tissues that both surround and support the teeth, maintaining them in the maxillary and mandibular bones. The word comes from the Greek terms peri-, meaning 'around' and -odons, meaning 'tooth.' Literally taken, it means that which is 'around the tooth'. Periodontics is the dental specialty that relates specifically to the care and maintenance of these tissues. The following four tissues make up the Periodontium: · Alveolar bone · Cementum

· Gingiva or gums

· Periodontal ligament

·

Prevalence	In epidemiology, the Prevalence of a disease in a statistical population is defined as the total number of cases of the disease in the population at a given time, or the total number of cases in the population, divided by the number of individuals in the population. It is used as an estimate of how common a condition is within a population over a certain period of time. It helps physicians or other health professionals understand the probability of certain diagnoses and is routinely used by epidemiologists, health care providers, government agencies and insurers.
Assessment	Educational Assessment is the process of documenting, usually in measurable terms, knowledge, skills, attitudes and beliefs. Assessment can focus on the individual learner, the learning community (class, workshop, or other organized group of learners), the institution, or the educational system as a whole. According to the Academic Exchange Quarterly: 'Studies of a theoretical or empirical nature addressing the Assessment of learner aptitude and preparation, motivation and learning styles, learning outcomes in achievement and satisfaction in different educational contexts are all welcome, as are studies addressing issues of measurable standards and benchmarks'.
Dental plaque	Dental plaque is biofilm (usually colorless) that builds up on the teeth. If not removed regularly by good oral hygiene measures, it can lead to dental cavities (caries) or periodontal problems .
	Plaque consists of microorganisms and extracellular matrix.
Biofilm	A biofilm is an aggregate of microorganisms in which cells are stuck to each other and/or to a surface. These adherent cells are frequently embedded within a self-produced matrix of extracellular polymeric substance (EPS). biofilm EPS, which is also referred to as 'slime,' is a polymeric jumble of DNA, proteins and polysaccharides.
Risk factor	In epidemiology, a Risk factor is a variable associated with an increased risk of disease or infection. Sometimes, determinant is also used, being a variable associated with either increased or decreased risk. Risk factors or determinants are correlational and not necessarily causal, because correlation does not imply causation.

Chapter 3. PART III: Chapter 21 - Chapter 30

Chlorhexidine	Chlorhexidine is a chemical antiseptic. It kills (is bactericidal to) both gram-positive and gram-negative microbes, although it is less effective with some gram-negative microbes. It is also bacteriostatic.
Dental caries	Dental caries is a disease wherein bacterial processes damage hard tooth structure (enamel, dentin, and cementum). These tissues progressively break down, producing Dental caries. Two groups of bacteria are responsible for initiating caries: Streptococcus mutans and Lactobacillus.
Infection	An Infection is the detrimental colonization of a host organism by a foreign species. In an Infection, the infecting organism seeks to utilize the host's resources to multiply, usually at the expense of the host. The infecting organism, or pathogen, interferes with the normal functioning of the host and can lead to chronic wounds, gangrene, loss of an infected limb, and even death.
Toothpaste	Toothpaste is a paste or gel dentifrice used with a toothbrush to clean and maintain the aesthetics and health of teeth. Toothpaste is used to promote oral hygiene: it can aid in the removal of dental plaque and food from the teeth, aid in the elimination and/or masking of halitosis and deliver active ingredients such as fluoride or xylitol to prevent tooth and gum disease (gingivitis). Some dentist recommendations include brushing your teeth at least twice a day, if not more.
Syringe	A Syringe is a simple piston pump consisting of a plunger that fits tightly in a tube. The plunger can be pulled and pushed along inside a cylindrical tube (the barrel), allowing the Syringe to take in and expel a liquid or gas through an orifice at the open end of the tube. The open end of the Syringe may be fitted with a hypodermic needle, a nozzle, or tubing to help direct the flow into and out of the barrel.
Periodontal disease	Periodontal diseases are those diseases that affect one or more of the periodontal tissues: · alveolar bone · periodontal ligament · cementum · gingiva

95

While many different diseases affect the tooth-supporting structures, plaque-induced inflammatory lesions make up the vast majority of Periodontal diseases and have traditionally been divided into two categories:

· gingivitis or

· periodontitis.

While in some sites or individuals, gingivitis never progresses to periodontitis, data indicates that gingivitis always precedes periodontitis.

Investigation into the causes and characteristics of Periodontal diseases began in the 18th century with pure clinical observation, and this remained the primary form of investigation well into the 19th century. During this time, the signs and symptoms of Periodontal diseases were firmly established:

· Rather than a single disease entity, Periodontal disease is a combination of multiple disease processes that share a common clinical manifestation.

· The etiology (cause) includes both local and systemic factors.

· The disease consists of a chronic inflammation associated with loss of alveolar bone.

· Advanced disease features include pus and exudates.

· Essential aspects of successful treatment of Periodontal disease include initial debridement and maintenance of proper oral hygiene.

Abscess	An abscess is a collection of pus (dead neutrophils) that has accumulated in a cavity formed by the tissue on the basis of an infectious process (usually caused by bacteria or parasites) or other foreign materials (e.g., splinters, bullet wounds, or injecting needles). It is a defensive reaction of the tissue to prevent the spread of infectious materials to other parts of the body.

The organisms or foreign materials kill the local cells, resulting in the release of cytokines.

Fluoride

Fluoride is the anion F⁻, the reduced form of fluorine. Both organic and inorganic compounds containing the element fluorine are sometimes called Fluorides. Fluoride, like other halides, is a monovalent ion (−1 charge).

Fluoride therapy

Fluoride therapy is the delivery of fluoride to the teeth topically or systemically in order to prevent tooth decay (dental caries) which results in cavities. Most commonly, fluoride is applied topically to the teeth using gels, varnishes, toothpaste/dentifrices or mouth rinse. Systemic delivery involves fluoride supplementation using water, salt, tablets or drops which are swallowed.

Osseointegration

Osseointegration is the direct structural and functional connection between living bone and the surface of a load-bearing artificial implant, typically made of titanium. It is a property virtually unique to titanium and hydroxylapatite, and has enhanced the science of medical bone, and joint replacement techniques.

In 1952, Prof.

Endodontic

Endodontics, from the Greek endo and odons (tooth), is one of the nine specialties of dentistry recognized by the American Dental Association, and deals with the tooth pulp and the tissues surrounding the root of a tooth. If the pulp (containing nerves, arterioles and venules as well as lymphatic tissue and fibrous tissue) has become diseased or injured, Endodontic treatment is required to save the tooth.

.

Pathogen

A Pathogen, 'I give birth to') an infectious agent, or more commonly germ, is a biological agent that causes disease to its host. There are several substrates and pathways whereby Pathogens can invade a host; the principal pathways have different episodic time frames, but soil contamination has the longest or most persistent potential for harboring a Pathogen.

The body contains many natural orders of defense against some of the common Pathogens in the form of the human immune system and by some 'helpful' bacteria present in the human body's normal flora.

Chapter 3. PART III: Chapter 21 - Chapter 30

Assessment	Educational Assessment is the process of documenting, usually in measurable terms, knowledge, skills, attitudes and beliefs. Assessment can focus on the individual learner, the learning community (class, workshop, or other organized group of learners), the institution, or the educational system as a whole. According to the Academic Exchange Quarterly: 'Studies of a theoretical or empirical nature addressing the Assessment of learner aptitude and preparation, motivation and learning styles, learning outcomes in achievement and satisfaction in different educational contexts are all welcome, as are studies addressing issues of measurable standards and benchmarks'.
Debridement	In oral hygiene and dentistry, Debridement refers to the removal of plaque and calculus that have accumulated on the teeth. Debridement in this case may be performed using ultrasonic instruments, which fracture the calculus, thereby facilitating its removal, as well as hand tools, including periodontal scaler and curettes, or through the use of chemicals such as hydrogen peroxide.
Interdental	Interdental consonants are produced by placing the blade of the tongue (the top surface just behind the tip of the tongue) against the upper incisors. This differs from a dental consonant in that the tip of the tongue is placed between the upper and lower front teeth, and therefore may articulate with both the upper and lower incisors, while a dental consonant is articulated with the tongue against the back of the upper incisors. interdental consonants may be transcribed with both a subscript and a superscript bridge, as [n̪ᵃɪ̯†], if precision is required, but it is more common to transcribe them as advanced alveolars, for example [n̠Ÿ].
Symptom	A Symptom is a departure from normal function or feeling which is noticed by a patient, indicating the presence of disease or abnormality. A Symptom is subjective, observed by the patient, and not measured. A Symptom may not be a malady, for example Symptoms of pregnancy.
Pericoronitis	Pericoronitis is a common problem in young adults with partial tooth impactions. It usually occurs within 17 to 24 years of age as it is when the third molars start erupting. It occurs when the tissue around the wisdom tooth has become inflamed because bacteria have invaded the area.
Periodontal disease	Periodontal diseases are those diseases that affect one or more of the periodontal tissues:

· alveolar bone

· periodontal ligament

· cementum

· gingiva

While many different diseases affect the tooth-supporting structures, plaque-induced inflammatory lesions make up the vast majority of Periodontal diseases and have traditionally been divided into two categories:

· gingivitis or

· periodontitis.

While in some sites or individuals, gingivitis never progresses to periodontitis, data indicates that gingivitis always precedes periodontitis.

Investigation into the causes and characteristics of Periodontal diseases began in the 18th century with pure clinical observation, and this remained the primary form of investigation well into the 19th century. During this time, the signs and symptoms of Periodontal diseases were firmly established:

· Rather than a single disease entity, Periodontal disease is a combination of multiple disease processes that share a common clinical manifestation.

· The etiology (cause) includes both local and systemic factors.

· The disease consists of a chronic inflammation associated with loss of alveolar bone.

· Advanced disease features include pus and exudates.

· Essential aspects of successful treatment of Periodontal disease include initial debridement and maintenance of proper oral hygiene.

AIDS

Acquired immune deficiency syndrome or acquired immunodeficiency syndrome (AIDS) is a disease of the human immune system caused by the human immunodeficiency virus (HIV).

This condition progressively reduces the effectiveness of the immune system and leaves individuals susceptible to opportunistic infections and tumors. HIV is transmitted through direct contact of a mucous membrane or the bloodstream with a bodily fluid containing HIV, such as blood, semen, vaginal fluid, preseminal fluid, and breast milk.

Root planing

The objective of scaling and root planing, otherwise known as conventional periodontal therapy or non-surgical periodontal therapy, is to remove or eliminate the etiologic agents which cause inflammation: dental plaque, its products and calculus, thus helping to establish a periodontium that is free of disease.

Periodontal scaling procedures 'include the removal of plaque, calculus and stain from the crown and root surfaces of teeth, whereas root planing is a specific treatment that removes the roughened cementum and surface dentin that is impregnated with calculus, microorganisms and their toxins.'

Scaling and root planing are often referred to as deep cleaning, and may be performed using a number of dental tools, including ultrasonic instruments and hand instruments, such as periodontal scalers and curettes.

Removal of adherent plaque and calculus with hand instruments can also be performed on patients without periodontal disease.

Premedication

Premedication refer to a drug treatment given to a patient before a (surgical or invasive) medical procedure. These drugs are typically sedative or analgesic.

Premedication before chemotherapy for cancer often refers to special drug regimens (usually 2 or more drugs, e.g.

Periodontitis	Periodontitis refers to a number of inflammatory diseases affecting the periodontium -- that is, the tissues that surround and support the teeth. periodontitis involves progressive loss of the alveolar bone around the teeth, and if left untreated, can lead to the loosening and subsequent loss of teeth. periodontitis is caused by microorganisms that adhere to and grow on the tooth's surfaces, along with an overly aggressive immune response against these microorganism.
Immunodeficiency	Immunodeficiency is a state in which the immune system's ability to fight infectious disease is compromised or entirely absent. Most cases of Immunodeficiency are acquired ('secondary') but some people are born with defects in the immune system, or primary Immunodeficiency. Transplant patients take medications to suppress their immune system as an anti-rejection measure, as do some patients suffering from an over-active immune system.

CPSIA information can be obtained at www.ICGtesting.com
Printed in the USA
243668LV00002B/369/P